My Life Is In Your Hands

A Nutritional Guide From
Birth to Adolescence

By Catherine Chapman

Dedicated to my children
Katrina and Evan with much love.

Published by Best Food Friends Pty Ltd.

First published in electronic form 2019.

Publication details
ISBN: 978-0-6482942-3-8
Chapman, Catherine, 1955-

My Life Is In Your Hands is exactly what we as nutrition professionals want to see being created for families. It provides facts and guidance that are sustainable for a parent to implement for years to come while raising a child. Nutrition can get confusing with new fad diets and social media, but the book sticks to the basics of how to properly fuel a child as they grow. 10 out of 10. Recommended for every parent!

Jourdan Mercurio-Lewis, MSNHP

Owner/Nutritionist of Summit Nutrition

Table of Contents

Introduction

Why It Is Important to Establish Healthy Eating Patterns in Our Children

If you are a parent, it is your specific responsibility to teach your child how to eat in a healthy and nutritious manner. This is because eating well when young is the best way to diminish the chances of illness, obesity, and learning difficulties later in life. And it's the best preventative medicine for avoiding them at any age. If you teach children how to eat well while they are young, they are less likely to grow up addicted to unhealthy, refined, sugary, overly salty, 'junk' foods devoid of nutrition.

Children who are taught healthy eating patterns from an early age will profit from good health, are more likely to remain fit, and will be less prone to diabetes, joint pain and immune disorders. They will be healthier because you, as their role model, will have taught them good nutrition and healthy eating habits as a form of preventative medicine early in life.

There are definite phases of growth that are part of "growing up", and each phase requires a different approach to eating and nutrition.

In this book we will discuss the following phases of human development:

- Newborn Eating Patterns (0–30 days)
- Infant Eating Patterns (1–12 months)
- Toddler Eating Patterns (1–3 years)
- Play Age Eating Patterns (4–9 years)
- Pre-teen Eating Patterns (10–12 years)
- Adolescent Eating Patterns (13–19 years)

In each chapter, we will also discuss:

- What to expect from a child of that age
- How many times a day to feed your child or teen
- Special nutritional needs of children at that age
- Challenges to eating well
- The best approaches to persuade children to eat well

Instilling healthy eating patterns in children can be a long and painstaking process. Media surrounding your children are constantly exposing them to all kinds of temptations that are unhealthy. And if you're on a tight schedule every day, it will be understandably difficult to implement a healthy eating routine. On top of that, there will inevitably be unhealthy influences from your children's friends and some parents who may ignore the benefits of healthy food choices.

As a general rule, you have to be a bit creative in your approach to convincing children of any age to eat in a healthy manner, to eat on a regular schedule and to love those foods that are good for them.

You will never regret the extra effort it takes to give your child this good, strong head start in life. It is a guarantee of good general health, strength, and a defence against illnesses, including cancers, immunity problems, mental health problems, and obesity.

Chapter 1: Newborn Eating Patterns

(0–30 Days Old)

What to Expect From Your Newborn

The eating patterns of a newborn baby can be summed up in one word: *Unpredictable.*

The bottom line is, at this age you are not going to be the one calling the shots when it comes to feeding. It is best to let Mother Nature take the lead. At this stage there are no real desires or thoughts that could be interfering with a child's need to eat, so it's simply pure instinct that makes the demand for food.

Be prepared to drop whatever it is you are doing, get up in the middle of the night, or do whatever it takes to feed your child any time it displays signs that he or she is hungry.

When a newborn is hungry, it may not necessarily cry or fuss around. Look for early signs of hunger, such as stirring and stretching, sucking motions, and lip movements.

Other cues that the baby is hungry are:

- Moving their heads from side to side
- Sticking out their tongues with a pushing motion
- Placing their fists in their mouths
- Puckering their lips
- Nuzzling against an arm or breast

It's also important, however, to realise that babies cry for reasons other than hunger. Sometimes babies just need to be cuddled or changed. They could also be over stimulated or too hot or cold.

One way to tell if your baby is, indeed, ready to eat is to check the clock. If your baby is crying only an hour after a recent feeding, it is likely that he or she is not really hungry but rather in distress for another reason.

It is also a good idea to make sure that the baby is not too full. When your baby stops sucking, closes his or her mouth, or turns away from the nipple or bottle, he or she may be satisfied or simply taking a break.

Try burping your baby or waiting a minute before offering food again. If your baby is ready to end the feeding session, he or she may dawdle or slow down the sucking of the nipple of the breast or bottle.

The brain has a mechanism that tells the body when to stop eating, and this mechanism is very much intact in healthy newborns. Staying in tune with your infant's subtle actions regarding satiety will keep you from trying to make the baby eat more because you think it might not have eaten enough. Some new parents believe, wrongly, that if they feed a baby more now, they won't have to feed it as often. It's a good idea not to feed a baby too much. This teaches it, on a primal and instinctual level, when to be satisfied, and those instincts will carry over later in life.

The healthiest thing that you can do for a newborn child is *feed-it-on-demand*. Be ready with the breast (or the bottle) at all times.

The Mayo Clinic recommends breastfeeding your child, as it offers a completely natural immunity straight from the mother. This is one way to give your child a really strong, healthy start in life.[1]

The Newborn Feeding Schedule

Most newborns require feeding eight to twelve times a day (or every two to three hours). This frantic need to eat slowly tapers off and the baby will likely be satisfied with six to eight feedings a day as time progresses.

One thing to keep in mind is that a breastfed baby may eat a little more often than one that is fed with formula. That is because breast milk moves a lot swifter through the baby's digestive system.[2]

Your baby won't necessarily eat the same amount every day. During growth spurts—often at 10 to 14 days after birth, as well as between three and six weeks—your baby may want more at each feeding, or want to be fed more often. After a few days, the pattern should become more predictable. When your baby begins to drop middle-of-the-night feedings, he or she may want a daytime "catch-up" feeding as well.

Newborn Feeding Challenges and Issues

The biggest controversy around feeding newborns is whether or not to breastfeed. There are situations in which it should be permissible to feed the baby formula instead of breast milk. One major reason for this is simply because the baby will not latch onto the breast and is therefore incapable of breastfeeding.

The American Academy of Pediatrics (AAP) joins other organisations such as the American Medical Association (AMA), the American Dietetic Association (ADA), and the World Health Organization (WHO) in recommending breastfeeding as the best option for newborn babies.[3]

Breastfeeding does have many challenges, but perhaps the most daunting one of all is the amount of time needed to feed a baby properly. The mother will find herself in demand every couple of hours. This can be very difficult for a woman who works, has to run errands, or travels. A baby drinking bottled formula needs to be fed less than a breastfed baby, so young mothers may see breastfeeding as a hassle.

Yet another challenge for some mothers who breastfeed might be the need to be careful what they eat and drink. What the mother eats can be passed through the breast milk to the child. If you do not want to be vigilant about what you consume, then breastfeeding is not for you.

Breastfeeding women should avoid fish that is high in mercury and wait at least two hours after drinking alcohol to avoid it being passed to the baby. If you do drink alcohol often, then you are doing your baby a favour by not breastfeeding, as any alcohol passed through your breast milk will be harmful to the baby.

Furthermore, breastfeeding mothers should also keep their caffeine intake to no more than one to three cups of coffee a day. Babies can absorb caffeine through breast milk and become addicted or irritable.[4]

The benefits to breastfeeding your child are great:

- Breastfed children have less diarrhoea[5]
- They are less likely to catch the flu virus as they age[6]
- Babies who are breastfed do not get as many inner-ear infections (See Endnote 6)
- Babies who are breastfed are less likely to die from SIDS (Sudden Infant Death Syndrome)[7]

- Children who have been breastfed are less likely to develop food allergies[8]
- Breastfed children are less likely to develop eczema[9]
- A study called "Breast Milk and Subsequent Intelligence Quotient in Children Born Preterm" in the *Lancet* found that breastfed babies are more intelligent[10]
- Breastfed children have healthier, stronger teeth[11]
- Breastfed babies tend to be less prone to developing diabetes[12]

Breast milk contains all kinds of nutrients and substances that simply cannot be found anywhere else. Whether breastfeeding or not, eventually your baby will fall into a fairly predictable feeding schedule of taking in more milk in less time at each feeding.

Alternating Breasts

There is also the issue of whether to alternate breasts when feeding a child. For years, mothers have been feeding newborns using one breast for five or ten minutes and then switching to the other breast. However, recently lactation specialists have started recommending that mothers *not* switch from one breast to another until the first is "empty". This allows the baby to receive more of the fattier and nutritious mother's milk known as "hind fat", which is at the end of the supply.

By the way, breastfeeding mothers tend to be healthier as well. It burns up to 500 calories a day and helps shrink the uterus, so your body returns to its pre-pregnancy shape faster.

According to a study at the National Institute of Health, giving your baby your own milk can also help reduce your chances of developing breast cancer, high blood pressure, diabetes and cardiovascular disease. It can also help decrease the risk of ovarian and uterine cancer.[13]

Is Your Newborn Full?

Newborns who are skinny may not actually be eating enough. Signs that your baby is satisfied are:

- The baby seems content and does not fuss constantly
- Produces between four to six soaked nappies a day
- Has regular bowel movements
- Is alert
- Is gaining weight
- Sleeps well at night

Your baby may therefore not be getting enough to eat if he or she does not appear to be satisfied after eating, is fussy, is not gaining weight, and is not creating several wet nappies a day.[14]

Special Nutritional Needs of Newborns

If you are feeding your newborn with breast milk, then there simply should be no need for any type of vitamin supplementation.

However, if you are feeding your baby formula milk, be sure to talk with your doctor about Vitamin D supplements for your baby (and possibly for yourself). Breast milk and formula may not provide enough Vitamin D, which is essential in helping your baby absorb the calcium and phosphorus necessary for strong bones. Too little Vitamin D may also cause rickets, a softening and weakening of the bones.

There are two points of view in place about whether or not you need to supplement a breastfed newborn baby's diet with Vitamin D.

The theory is that, if the mother has not had enough sun exposure or Vitamin D during her pregnancy, then the newborn baby's diet of breast milk should be supplemented. Vitamin D can be synthesised quite simply by the baby when the sun shines on his or her skin.

If you live in a southern climate, where there is not much sun or where you experience a long winter, then the baby may need supplementation. In northern climates, limit the newborn's exposure to the point where the skin just begins to turn pink; about twenty minutes. After that, apply sunscreen for longer periods in the sun, but do not completely deny your baby sunlight.

At midday, the sun is at its highest point and UVB rays are the most intense. This is the best time to get the needed vitamin D. But be careful. Your baby's skin is not accustomed to intense sun yet, so keep a diligent eye out for skin turning slightly pink, then cover baby up. Additionally, when the sun is lower than 50 degrees above the horizon, you will be exposed to the more dangerous UVA rays. This is when it's also important to cover your baby's skin with clothing or stay in the shade.[15]

Why Formula is Not the Best Food

Breastfed infants tend to be better nourished. Breast milk contains lactose, protein and fat and is easily digested by a newborn's immature system. Also, none of the naturally occurring important antibodies found in breast milk are found in manufactured formula, which means that formula doesn't provide the baby with the added protection against infection and illness that breast milk does.

Although breastfeeding is recommended, there are some women who are unable to provide natural milk to their child for varied reasons.

Food Standards Australian and New Zealand (FSANZ) and the US Food and Drug Administration (FDA) regulate formula companies to ensure that they provide all the known necessary nutrients (including Vitamin D) in their formulas.

Commercial formulas are coming closer to duplicating what is in a new mother's milk but have yet to match the exact combination and composition. The substances in breast milk are currently too complex to identify and imitate exactly.

If you are going to feed your baby with formula, you need to make sure that you boil the water before you mix it. It is important that it is sterile. You also need to sterilise bottles and nipples to avoid transferring bacteria to your baby.

Never store a bottle of formula in a refrigerator for longer than two hours and never feed your baby bottled formula that has been left out for more than one hour. You can make your baby very sick if you ignore these rules.

How to Convince Your Child to Suckle

A newborn who seems to be fussing and unable to enjoy eating may have issues around food later in life. The baby could become a picky eater or simply have bad associations with eating and end up being underweight.

It is essential that your baby "latch" on to the breast and learn how to suckle as part of a routine that teaches him or her to have a positive attitude towards food.

The basis of breastfeeding is getting the baby to latch on well. A baby who latches on well gets milk well. A baby who latches on poorly has more difficulty getting milk, therefore will be hungrier and gain less weight. A baby who feels secure and comfortable in your arms has a better chance of getting optimum nutrition from breastfeeding.

Try rocking the baby in your arms or sitting in a rocking chair. Support your back and arms with a pillow, if necessary, so that both of you feel stable and are not shifting around.

There are quite a few other ways you can convince your baby to suckle even if he or she is reluctant.

- Give your baby lots of attention and skin-to-skin contact.
- Nurse without a bra.
- Nurse the baby when he or she is sleepy. (You will be more successful if you feed while he or she is drifting off or just starting to wake up.)
- Minimise distractions by nursing in a dark quiet room.

Studies have also shown that having the two of you in the same room at night can create a bond that also makes feeding at the breast more relaxing and positive for the child.[16]

If you are having trouble getting your baby to latch on, you can get a consultation with a lactation expert. Do not be afraid to get this advice. Most maternity and neonatal care departments have a lactation expert on staff to specifically help women having issues with breastfeeding.

Top Ten Tips for Feeding Newborns

1. Do not try to force your baby to eat according to your schedule. It is simply not going to happen. For a healthy baby, be sure to feed him or her when they're hungry. Feed your baby on demand.

2. Be aware of your newborn's silent signals that he or she is hungry, such as: lip puckering, nuzzling and suckling on his or her own fist. Too much frustration around feedings can lead to unhealthy relationships with eating and insecurities later in life.

3. Breastfeeding a baby is always preferable as mother's milk contains everything a baby needs to grow up healthy. This also means that your baby will mature into an individual who does not have trouble with basic bodily functions and will be as healthy as possible.

4. Alternate breasts when breastfeeding so that the baby receives the more nutritious "hind milk", which is at the end. Don't make your baby change sides during feeding; wait until he or she has finished before offering the other breast.

5. Don't overfeed a baby. Know that not every cry or complaint is because of hunger. A spoiled baby is one that may learn to use food as emotional blackmail or reward, which can be frustrating for the mother and unhealthy for the baby.

6. Be sure to ask your doctor about whether or not your newborn needs supplementation with Vitamin D. A deficiency is detrimental to bone development.

7. If you are feeding your baby with a bottle, be sure that all water you prepare formulas with is absolutely sterile. Giving your baby bad water can be life threatening.

8. Never store a bottle of formula in a refrigerator for longer than two hours and never feed your baby bottled formula that has been left out at room temperature for more than one hour.

9. Be as relaxed as possible when feeding the baby. Support yourself with a pillow or rock back and forth in a rocking chair. A comfortable, relaxed mother is encouraging to a newborn baby.

10. Studies suggest that mothers and babies sleeping in the same room during the first month of birth are more relaxed, better bonded, and better able to breastfeed. This helps develop a positive attitude towards food because the experience of eating has not been a stressful time.

Chapter 2: Infant Eating Patterns

(1–12 Months Old)

What to Expect From Your Baby During the First Year

Once your baby reaches the one-month stage, he or she is no longer a 'newborn'. The proper name for a baby from one month to one year old is 'baby' or 'infant'.

After the baby is one month old, you might notice some changes in his or her behaviour. The baby may respond more to your voice and objects, and may give you more cues that he or she is hungry. Crying persistently until fed might become more of a pattern.

Once your baby is approximately four months old, he or she might be able to eat soft baby food. You do not have to rush to give babies solid food; each baby is different.

The baby will be mobile and crawling at approximately six months, and at that point may be more interested in eating solid foods.

Between six and twelve months, your baby will be developing motor skills and verbal skills that have him or her groping or grasping for food, and if the child is very advanced, actually requesting favourite menu items in "baby talk".

Between nine and twelve months, your baby may become more distractible and less interested in food. This is a good sign, because it means the baby's internal organs are developing normally and that he or she can subsist on less food.

The Infant Feeding Schedule

It is important to remember that every baby is different and that what follows constitutes a rough guideline of what to expect as the baby develops.

One to Four Months

Feed your baby breast milk or formula only. Your baby's digestive tract is still developing so solid food is not an option just yet.

- From 1–2 months old, a baby should be fed between 60 and 120 ml, 6 to 8 times, every 24 hours.
- From 2–3 months old, a baby should be fed between 150 and 180 ml, 5 to 6 times, every 24 hours.
- From 3–6 months old, a baby should be fed between 180 and 210 ml, 5 to 6 times, every 24 hours.

Four to Six Months

Your infant is ready for solid food when:

- He or she can hold her head up
- Sit up in a high chair
- Can close his or her mouth around a spoon
- Can move food from the front to back of mouth
- Seems hungry after eight to ten feedings of breast milk

At this stage, you will be feeding your baby a combination of breast milk and formula, plus his or her first pureed foods.[17]

Good introductory pureed foods to feed your child are: sweet potatoes, squash, apples, bananas, peaches or pears.

The very first food you should feed your child is an iron-rich instant cereal. Begin with about 1 teaspoon of pureed food or cereal. Mix cereal with 4 to 5 teaspoons of breast milk or formula.

By around four to six months of age, birth stores of iron are becoming depleted and an outside source becomes necessary. Establishing a baby on an iron-fortified cereal will help secure their iron status throughout infancy and toddlerhood, when it is most significant.[18]

Increase to 1 tablespoon of pureed food or 1 tablespoon of cereal mixed with breast milk or formula twice a day. If giving cereal, gradually thicken the consistency by using less liquid.

If you are not sure exactly when to introduce solid foods to your baby, one rule of thumb is that the baby is typically ready when his or her present weight is double their birth weight.[19]

Six to Eight Months

At this age, your baby will still be drinking breast milk or formula but should also be eating:

- Iron-fortified rice, barley or oat cereals (rice, barley, oats)
- Pureed or strained fruits (banana, pears, apples, peaches)
- Pureed or strained vegetables (stewed carrots, squash, sweet potato)

- Pureed meat (chicken, pork, beef, lamb)
- Pureed tofu
- Pureed legumes (black beans, chickpeas, soybeans, broad beans, black-eyed peas, lentils, kidney beans)

The amounts per day should be:

- 3–9 tablespoons of cereal in two to three feedings
- 1 teaspoon to half a cup of fruit in two or three feedings
- 1 teaspoon of vegetables increased to half a cup in two or three feedings

It is best to introduce new foods one at a time, with at least three days in between meals to make sure your baby is not allergic.[20]

Eight to Ten Months

At this age, the baby is able to pick up objects and grasp them and transfer food from one hand to another. This is also the age at which your baby will start to put everything in his or her mouth to see what it tastes like.

Your baby will still be on formula, but solid foods and finger foods should be more prominent in the diet.

At eight to ten months you can start feeding your baby:

- Small amounts of soft cheese, yogurt, cottage cheese
- Iron-fortified cereals (rice, barley, wheat, oats, mixed cereals)
- Mashed fruits and vegetables (bananas, peaches, pears, avocados, cooked carrots, squash, potatoes, sweet potatoes)

- Finger foods (lightly toasted bread pieces, chunks of ripe banana, well-cooked spiral pasta, teething rusks)
- Small amounts of protein (egg, pureed meats, poultry, boneless fish, tofu, well-cooked mashed lentils, split peas, pinto beans, black beans)

The optimum breakdown of these foods should be:

- 1/4 to 1/3 cup dairy (or approximately 15 grams of cheese)
- 1/4 to 1/2 cup iron-fortified cereal
- 1/4 to 1/2 cup fruit
- 1/4 to 1/2 cup vegetables
- 1/8 to 1/4 cup protein foods

Once again, be sure to introduce foods gradually with at least three days in between each new sampling to make sure your baby is not allergic.

Try to avoid infant feeders. These syringe-like gadgets basically force-feed solids into infants. A normal baby will never need this. Either he or she is too young to take food from a spoon (thus doesn't need the solids yet anyway) or he or she can take some off a spoon, even if it doesn't seem like "enough".

Ten to Twelve Months

At this age, the baby has more teeth, swallows food with more ease, and may be trying to use a spoon.

Aside from breast milk, babies at this age can also have:

- Soft pasteurised cheese, yogurt, cottage cheese
- Iron-fortified cereals (rice, barley, wheat, oats, mixed cereals)
- Fruit cut into cubes or strips, or mashed

- Bite-size, soft-cooked vegetables (peas, carrots)
- Combo foods (macaroni and cheese, casseroles)
- Protein (eggs pureed or finely ground meats, poultry, and boneless fish, tofu, well-cooked and mashed beans)
- Finger foods (lightly toasted bread or bagels, small pieces of ripe banana, spiral pasta, teething rusks)

The amounts that are healthy are:

- 1/3 cup dairy (or approximately 15 grams of cheese)
- 1/4 to 1/2 cup iron-fortified cereal
- 1/4 to 1/2 cup fruit
- 1/4 to 1/2 cup vegetables
- 1/8 to 1/4 cup combo foods
- 1/8 to 1/4 cup protein foods

At this point, you might find that your baby is eating a little less. This is completely normal. It means that your baby's digestive system is in full development.

Although your baby will become more dexterous and have a better gag reflex, avoid foods that are potential choking hazards like grapes, peanuts and nuts.

Eating at the same time every day will also help your baby adapt to eating solid food.

Baby Feeding Challenges and Issues

One of the biggest challenges of feeding a baby under one year old is knowing when he or she is actually ready for solid food.

If you feed a baby solid food too early, there is a risk that he or she will develop a food allergy or be unable to digest the food. The result can be ongoing stomach problems and bowel disorders.

This is why it is so important to err on the side of caution and make sure the baby is ready to eat solid food. If you are really unsure, ask the advice of your doctor.

While still breastfeeding, it is also very important for a mother to avoid spicy foods as these can pass through the breast milk and cause vomiting, diarrhoea, and stomach pain. Also, if you do not want a 'gassy' baby, then stay away from gas-producing foods such as broccoli and cabbage.

Another issue is whether or not you should serve your child commercially bought baby food. While it is fast and convenient, commercial baby food may not be as fresh or nutritious (or cost effective) as home-made baby food.

It is also very important for you to check the ingredients on any commercial food to make sure that they do not contain any of the following additives.

Additives to Avoid in Baby Food

If you buy baby food with additives in it, you may be addicting your baby to fats, sugars, preservatives and many other unhealthy things for life. Many commercial baby foods contain additives to make them look and taste better, or to add to shelf life.

The side effects of babies eating foods that are unhealthy for them include: food allergies, increased waistlines, an inability to absorb minerals and vitamins, a fatty liver, childhood obesity, learning and behavioural disabilities, and many different childhood cancers and diseases.

To avoid introducing babies to a lifetime pattern of unhealthy eating habits, here is a breakdown of the types of foods you simply must avoid.

Artificial Sweeteners

These are combinations of chemicals that make food taste sweeter. Beware of finding them in baby foods that are labelled 'natural', 'sugar-free' or 'organic'.

These sweeteners encourage cravings for more sweeteners and train the brain to crave calorie-high, artificial foods. Many foods that contain artificial sweeteners are also of poor nutritional quality.

To avoid establishing an unhealthy taste for sweets in your infant, Splenda should be avoided, along with Saccharin, NutraSweet, and Sweet N'Low.[21]

Monosodium Glutamate (MSG)

Monosodium Glutamate can be toxic for infants. It is used to bring out the flavour in foods and although, thankfully, it is not present in most current baby foods any more, you should still read the labels and watch out for it. Beware of any ingredient called "spices" as this can be MSG.

If you are pureeing your own baby food, be sure to watch out for pickled foods and condiments that might contain MSG.

MSG may also be hidden in infant formula, low-fat milk, lollies, chewing gum, drinks and over-the-counter medications (especially children's cold medicines).[22]

Children are four times more sensitive to MSG than adults. Neonatal exposure to MSG can cause a permanent reduction in the secretion of growth hormone, leading to stunted growth and irreversible obesity.

Other reactions to MSG include: headaches, nausea, weakness, a burning sensation in the back of neck and forearms, wheezing, changes in heart rate and difficulty breathing.

Artificial Colours

Artificial colours do not occur naturally. Many are made from coal tar and can contain up to ten parts per million of arsenic and lead and still be approved by the US FDA. FSANZ in Australia says that this level is safe but do warn that children can have allergic reactions.

Artificial colours can cause allergic reactions, hyperactivity and ADD (Attention Deficit Disorder) in children. They may contribute to visual and learning disorders or cause nerve damage. The use of colouring in products normally indicates that other natural ingredients that may contain the colour, like oranges, have not been used.

Here is a list of the **worst colouring agents**.

Blue #1, found in baked goods, lollies and soft drinks, has been shown to damage the chromosomes in a cell's nucleus and cause retardation in both children and adults.

Blue #2, which is found in lollies, may cause brain tumours.

Citrus Red #1, is sprayed on green oranges to make them look ripe, so even if you are making juice or puree for your baby, you could be giving him or her a poisonous chemical additive that causes cancer. Always make sure your produce is organic.

Citrus Red #2, used to colour the skins of some Florida oranges, can cause cancer if the peel is eaten.

Red #3, is often added to canned cherry pie filling, maraschino cherries, baked goods, and ice cream. Studies have linked this dye to nerve damage and thyroid cancer.

Red #40, is found in soft drinks, lollies, gelatin desserts, pastry, pet food, and sausage, and is a suspected carcinogen.

Yellow #5, is the second most widely used colourant and it contributes to behavioural disturbances in children and can cause allergic reactions. It is found in gelatin desserts and baked goods.

Yellow #6, can cause tumours in the adrenal glands and kidneys. It is found in beverages, sausage, baked goods, lollies, and gelatin (See Endnote 22.)

BHA and BHT

These are preservatives that are found in baby food. They stop food oils from going rancid. These additives seem to affect sleep and appetite and have been associated with liver and kidney damage, baldness, behavioural problems, cancer, foetal abnormalities, and growth retardation.

Sodium Nitrate and Nitrite

These are preservatives that are added to processed meat products such as bacon, corned beef, ham, hot dogs, lunch meats, and sausage. They prevent the growth of bacteria.

They are considered dangerous by the Therapeutic Goods Administration, but they have not been banned because they prevent botulism.

Side effects of eating these preservatives include: headaches, nausea, vomiting, and dizziness. You may find them in baby foods that contain meat, so be sure to read labels before you buy commercially made food.

Partially Hydrogenated Vegetable Oil

Partially hydrogenated vegetable oil is difficult to avoid and is found in a lot of baby foods. It is one of the main justifications as to why you just might want to make your own baby food.

Trans fats can be found in foods such as vegetable shortening, some margarines, crackers, lollies, baked goods, biscuits and cookies, snack foods, fried foods, salad dressings and many processed foods. They are associated with heart disease, breast and colon cancer, atherosclerosis and elevated cholesterol.

A word of warning: if the list of ingredients on a package is long, there are probably a lot of chemical additives in the product. It's best to avoid these foods, not only because of the individual effects of the additives, but also because of the unknown health effects of combinations of food additives. (See Endnote 22.)

Keep in mind that you might want to stay away from these additives in any food that you buy for children of any age.

The best way to avoid all of this, is to simply make your own baby food. A baby can eat any food that you can puree or process in a blender, including the nutritious meals that you might be making for older members of your family.

Foods That Are Choking Hazards

Avoid giving your baby any foods that are choking hazards.

- Large chunks of cut up fruit.
- Round fruits like grapes, cherry tomatoes, and melon balls.
- Soft sticky foods like marshmallows or gummy lollies that can get lodged in the throat.

Remember that an infant under one year just simply does not have the glottis, oesophagus or throat muscles needed to process these foods.

Special Nutritional Needs of Babies

Between the ages of four months and one year, there are some foods that should be avoided. This is true of these foods regardless of whether you are buying them commercially or trying to puree them while making your own home-made baby food.

Eggs

Babies from 1 month to a year old should ONLY eat egg yolk as egg white can be highly allergenic.

Cow's Milk

Your baby cannot digest the protein in cow's milk in their first year. Feeding your child cow's milk can damage his or her kidneys.

Soy Milk

Introducing soy milk to your child in the first year can create a soy allergy. It can also damage his or her kidneys.

Honey

Honey sounds like a health food but it is exactly the opposite for an infant.

Honey can contain spores of Clostridium botulinum, which causes botulism. An adult's intestinal tract can prevent the growth of these spores, but in a baby the spores can grow and produce life-threatening toxins.[23]

A Word About Pesticides

Shortly we will be discussing making home-made baby food. Every year more than two billion pounds of pesticides enter our environment. Yet only 10% of the pesticides approved for use on food have been adequately tested for use in humans.

Pesticides disable our ability to fight off infectious organisms and may impair fertility or contribute to miscarriages and birth defects.

Children tend to eat a limited number of foods, which can increase their exposure to specific pesticides. They also eat more food relative to their body weight than adults do, so they will get bigger doses of pesticides, despite the fact they are eating tinier amounts of food.

Children may also absorb pesticides more easily, and because their gastrointestinal tract is still developing, their bodies may be less capable of breaking them down.

Finally, pesticides can block the absorption of nutrients that are vital to healthy growth and development.

To protect your baby from eating pesticides in store-bought food or food that you are pureeing to make home-made food, you should take the following precautions.

- Peel fruits and vegetables and remove the outer leaves of vegetables like lettuce and cabbage.
- Scrub unpeeled vegetables under running water as thoroughly as possible.
- For foods that are more difficult to wash, like strawberries, grapes, broccoli, lettuce, and spinach, soak them briefly, then rinse them a few times.
- Stay away from produce that has mould, bruising, and decay. These are likely to harbour more pesticides.
- Trim animal fat from meat. Some pesticides (and other environmental chemicals) are concentrated in the fat and skin of poultry, meat and fish.
- Take the skin off chicken. Chicken skin absorbs pesticides from the grain chickens are fed.
- Look for locally grown produce. Fruit and vegetables that are grown far away require after-harvest pesticides and waxes to help them survive the long trip to the grocery store.
- Purchase produce in season. Out of season food usually comes from another hemisphere and has more pesticides

According to the US Environmental Working Group, the foods that contain **the highest levels of pesticides** in the United States are: celery, peaches, strawberries, apples, blueberries, nectarines, bell peppers, spinach, cherries, kale, cabbage leaves, potatoes, and imported grapes.

The foods that have **the lowest pesticide residues** are: onions, avocados, sweet corn, pineapple, mangos, sweet peas, asparagus, kiwi fruit, cabbage, eggplant, rock melon, watermelon, grapefruit, sweet potatoes, and honeydew melon.[24]

Stay Away from Genetically Modified Foods

Genetically Modified Organisms (GMOs) are plants and animals that have been genetically tampered with to try and develop a superior product, but they're not always marked as such. Some manufacturers will add "No GMOs" to their label.

In the US, the majority of the corn, soybean, cotton and canola crops are now genetically modified, and one or more of these crops can be found in nearly every processed food. There is no mandatory safety testing done by the FDA on GMOs.

Testing that has been done in the past has shown GMOs can increase food toxicity, allergy susceptibility, immune suppression, resistance to antibiotics and the incidence of cancer. (See Endnote 22.)

Buy Organic

A 2003 University of Washington study found that children who ate a diet of organic food had a level of pesticides in their bodies that was six times lower than children who ate ordinary food.

Many studies also show that organic fruits and vegetables are more nutritious; containing more

Vitamin C and antioxidants, which may help prevent heart disease and any number of other disorders.

A 2003 study at the University of California at Davis, for example, found that organic fruit has up to 58 percent more antioxidants than non-organic fruit.

Be careful when shopping for baby food. Unless a baby food specifically states that it is "certified organic", it may contain pesticides.

If you have the outdoor space, you might consider growing some of your own organic fruits and vegetables. Look for organic growers at your local farmers market, farm stand, or food cooperative. Most grocery stores now have organic produce sections. (See Endnote 24.)

Keep Sugar Out of Your Baby Food

High consumption of sugar and the corresponding elevated insulin levels can cause weight gain, bloating, fatigue, arthritis, migraines, lowered immune function, gallstones, obesity, breast cancer, gum disease, cavities, and cardiovascular disease. It can also prevent children's bodies from absorbing the B vitamins, calcium, magnesium, chromium and copper.

Children who eat lots of sugar actually eat significantly lower amounts of protein, and have decreased amounts of B vitamins, iron, zinc, and Vitamin E.

Be sure to read labels before you buy, because sugar comes in many disguises and has many names: dextrose, glucose, fructose, lactose, corn syrup, high-fructose corn syrup, maple sugar, honey, invert sugar, maltose, diastase, sorbitol, caramel, date sugar, dextran, fruit juice, fruit juice concentrate, ethyl maltol, maltodextrin, sorghum syrup, and more. (See Endnote 22.)

The Most Nutritious Foods for Baby

There are lots of healthy, baby-friendly foods out there, but some provide maximum nutritional value for minimal calorie and fat intake.

The idea is that the younger your children are when you start these foods, the more willing they will be to make these foods their favourites throughout life.

Here are some great ideas for making pureed baby food out of these nutritious foods.

Squash: Squash is an excellent source of Vitamins A and C, is naturally sweet, and has a pleasing, creamy texture. Roast the squash first and then sprinkle a little parmesan cheese on it or mix it with cooked and pureed chickpeas for a tasty combination.

Lentils: Lentils are protein and fibre rich. Combine cooked lentils with vegetables and rice.

Dark green leafy vegetables: Leafy greens boast high amounts of iron and folate. While spinach is perhaps the best known of this group, there are many other varieties, including: kale, silver beet, and cabbage leaves. Steam these greens and mix with a fortified cereal or a lean meat to make your baby a super power-packed nutritious food.

Broccoli: Brimming with folate, fibre, and calcium, steamed broccoli with a bit of parmesan cheese pleases most babies. Gnawing on pieces of chilled broccoli can also help soothe a teething baby.

Avocados: Avocados are wonderful when pureed with bananas or yams. They contain the essential fatty acids that assist your baby with brain development.

Blueberries: The deep brilliant blue of these berries comes from flavonoids called anthocyanins, which are good for your baby's eyes, brain, and urinary tract. Puree berries and swirl with breast milk or plain yogurt. They also go well with apples or canned salmon.

Meat: Meat is a good source of protein, B vitamins, and zinc. Make stew and then blend it up with a bit of ginger and parsley.

Prunes: Prunes have lots of fibre and can help your baby stay regular. Puree them and serve them straight or mixed in with cereal or apple sauce for a sweet treat.

Chickpeas: Like lentils and other beans, chickpeas are rich in protein and fibre and are delicious cooked with a bit of olive oil and then pureed.

Sweet Potatoes: Roast these with some olive oil and parsley and puree for a delicious, nutritious treat.[25]

How to Persuade Your Baby to Eat Solid Foods

A baby can become attached to drinking formula, and it can be hard for some children to be persuaded to start eating solid foods. On the other hand, it can seem like the baby is showing a lot of curiosity and wants to start eating solid foods like the rest of the family.

There is no medical evidence to show that feeding one food to your baby and not others is going to benefit the child. Recommended foods to start with include:

pureed sweet potatoes, squash, apple sauce, bananas, peaches, and pears.

To gently lead your baby into the idea of eating, nurse or bottle-feed him or her first. Then give the baby one or two teaspoons of pureed solid food.

If you decide to start with cereal, mix it with enough formula or breast milk to make a semi-liquid. Use a soft-tipped plastic spoon when you feed your baby to avoid injuring his or her gums.

If your baby doesn't seem very interested in eating off the spoon, let them smell and taste the food, or wait until they seem to want it.

Begin by feeding solid food once a day. Don't bother if the baby is too tired and cranky; he or she will simply not be up to the idea of doing anything outside his or her normal routine.

Your baby may not eat much in the beginning, but give him or her time to come around to the experience. Some babies need practice keeping food in their mouths and swallowing.

Once your baby becomes familiar with his or her new diet, they should be ready for a few tablespoons of food a day. If he or she is eating cereal, gradually thicken the consistency by adding less liquid. As the amount your baby eats increases, add another feeding until he or she can handle a mouthful.

Yes, your baby will need breast milk or formula until he or she is one year old. Both types of food provide important vitamins, iron and protein in an easy-to-digest form. Solid food can't replace all the nutrients that breast milk or formula provides during that first year.[26]

Babies not wanting to eat solid food may respond to eating fruit puree. This is only recommended if it has been a number of months and your baby is still not on solid food and refuses to eat cereals.

However, it can be a mistake to offer your baby fruit puree before vegetable puree. The baby may prefer to eat the fruit because it's naturally sweeter and just reject the vegetables.[27]

If you're offering a sippy cup at a young age, it's best to fill it with the liquid your baby is most familiar with. Either pumped breast milk or formula can be served in a cup, and a familiar taste will make your child more likely to want to get at what's in the cup. Some parents use juice as a bribe to encourage use of the cup, however, this can lead to your baby expecting to get juice every time he or she sees a cup.

The first time you offer your child a sippy cup, you might want to keep a bottle handy too just in case your child refuses the cup or takes only a small amount before rejecting it.

Choose an easy to grip cup with a lid that stays on securely. Twist-on lids are the best choice because they are more difficult for your child to take off. Look for cups that aren't too wide so that your child's little hands can hold it easily.

As with all transitions, learning to drink from a sippy cup can take some time. Be patient. Soon your child will be taking all liquids from a cup and the bottle will be a thing of the past.[28]

Top Ten Tips for Feeding Infants

1. Remember that every baby develops in a different way and that it may take some individuals longer to be able to eat solid food or sit up and use a spoon. There is no real "schedule"; do not stress your baby by forcing him or her into developmental stages (such as drinking from a sippy cup) before he or she is ready.

2. Mixing pureed food with a bit of formula can help a baby become familiar with solid food faster and with less indigestion. However, do not do this until the child is older than four months or he or she could develop food allergies.

3. Never force a child to eat or he/she may think eating is about "control". This could result in future insecurities about food. Offer the baby food and let him or her play with it.

4. Stick with fresh, brightly coloured vegetables whenever you can as they are loaded with the most vitamins and nutrients.

5. Eating at the same time every day and developing a routine helps your baby adjust to solid food.

6. Babies from one month to one year old should ONLY eat egg yolk as egg white can be highly allergenic.

7. Talk to your baby to make mealtimes seem more exciting and sociable. This will help the child develop a positive attitude toward food.

8. Try to avoid infant feeders. These syringe-like gadgets basically force-feed solids into infants. A normal baby will never need this. Either he/she is too young to take food from a spoon (and so doesn't need the solids yet anyway) or he/she can take

some off a spoon, even if it doesn't seem like "enough".

9. Avoid buying commercial baby foods that contain additives, colouring agents and toxic preservatives. Read the labels well.

10. Make your own fresh baby food from raw organic vegetables or cooked organic meat and serve it to your baby as much as possible to make sure he or she does not develop a taste for sugar, salt and other unhealthy foods.

Chapter 3: Toddler Eating Patterns

(1–3 Years Old)

What to Expect From Your Toddler

The first three years of life are a period of incredible growth in all areas of a baby's development.

Be sure to read this chapter no matter how old your child is. A lot of information in this chapter applies to children and also adults, especially in the nutrition sections.

From one year to two years old, the child will learn how to feed him or herself many different foods. You might also see the toddler begin to use utensils such as a fork or spoon. The toddler will be using actions and words to communicate thoughts and feelings. Your toddler may be showing you what he or she wants to eat, what he or she finds delicious, and what he or she does not want to eat.

You might find the child is more willing to try new foods and be more dependent on himself/herself instead of you.

The toddler is also going to start becoming quite messy. They love to play with their food and paint everything with it, including the tray and you. Many toddlers will throw food and plates for fun and also drop food on the floor.

From two years to three years old, the toddler might start choosing which foods to eat. He or she might use words to express thoughts and feelings.

This is the age at which your toddler will learn how to tell you he or she is full. This is very important in the long term. Knowing when to stop eating stops your toddler from growing up to be overweight.

Pay attention when your toddler makes a fuss about eating a certain food. It could be that the food is too strong in taste, too hot, or even that your toddler is having a mild allergic reaction to it.

A happy toddler is not screaming, crying, and protesting while eating. He or she may play with the food but usually they see mealtime as a positive, even creative experience.

Understanding that your toddler needs to play with food helps them develop in a healthy way later in life.

The Toddler Eating Schedule

From one to three years old, your toddler's palate will expand and so will your menu.

- Offer 3–4 healthy choices during mealtimes
- Offer 2–3 healthy snacks a day
- Stop making separate meals for the toddler and integrate what the whole family is eating into the toddler's diet

One of the most important things you can do for a toddler is to eat at the same time every day. This helps them get used to the idea of mealtime.

Yet another thing to expect is a restless toddler. Do not plan to have a child below three years old sit down with you and sit for too long. Keep mealtimes for the toddler about ten to twenty minutes long. A snacking session should not be longer than ten minutes.

It is also healthy to have the toddler eat with the rest of the family whenever possible so he or she becomes socialised.[29]

Special Nutritional Needs of Toddlers

Toddlers still eat baby food, so it's a good idea to re-read 'Special Nutritional Needs of Babies' in Chapter 2. In that chapter, additives and foods to avoid are outlined as well as specific guidelines for making delicious, nutritious baby foods.

In general, avoid:

- Sugar
- Too much salt
- MSG
- Cow's milk
- Additives
- Pesticides
- Overly spicy food

... and serve your child organic foods whenever possible.

Many of the fruits and vegetables mentioned in the chapter can also be sliced up into small chunks to make finger foods for the toddler to eat.

Toddlers tend to be quite active, especially if they are about to reach that age known as the "Terrible Twos". You should be quite careful not to give your child more than half a cup of juice a day. Even juice that is squeezed at home by you can contain a great deal of natural sugar. Your child can be temporarily pumped up by a surge of sugar then experience a terrible crash and become very cranky or miserable. If your little one seems to have a mood disorder, the culprit could actually be sugar.

The following are the American Academy of Pediatrics' guidelines on giving juice to young children.

- Parents need to know the difference between 100% fruit juice and juice drinks, beverages or cocktails, which may contain very little or no real fruit juice. These drinks can look like fruit juice, but are just as harmful as drinking a soft drink.
- Fruit juice should not be given to infants before 6 months of age.
- To help prevent tooth decay, children should not drink juice from bottles or cups that allow them to consume juice easily throughout the day.
- Babies and toddlers should not drink fruit juice at bedtime.
- For children ages 1 to 6, intake of fruit juice should be limited to one half to three quarters of a cup per day.
- Drinking too much juice can lead to poor nutrition, diarrhoea, gas, abdominal pain, bloating, and tooth decay.
- All children should be encouraged to eat whole fruits rather than drink juices.[30]

Once a baby becomes a toddler, he or she may suddenly be thirsty more often. This is because babies do not have as much need for water as the growing toddler does. Make sure your toddler is well hydrated throughout the day.

According to the US Institute of Medicine, a child between the ages of one and three needs about 1.3

litres of water a day. Since their body weight is much less than those of adults, toddlers can become dehydrated easily; they also tend to ignore their thirst while caught up in play.

If your toddler is not drinking enough water, dilute juice with equal parts of water before giving it to them. A fresh lemon or orange squeezed into half a glass of water with a pinch of sugar is another healthy alternative. Coconut water is a nutritious option.

By the time your child realises he or she is thirsty, they may already be mildly dehydrated, and they will most probably only ask for water once he or she feels tired or a bit dizzy. This could be especially true during hot weather.[31]

One thing you really do need to avoid is making formula or baby food with well water. *Formula and food prepared with water from a well can cause nitrate poisoning.*[32]

Issues and Challenges of Feeding Toddlers

Toddlers can be difficult, and they can throw tantrums. They do not have fully developed emotions or brains and can be very irrational little creatures.

Realise that being a picky eater is part of being a toddler. There are good reasons why kids between one and three years of age peck and poke at their food. After a year of rapid growth (the average one-year-old has tripled his or her birth weight), toddlers gain weight more slowly. So, of course, they need less food to support their system.

Toddlers sometime like to binge on one food at a time for days and then switch to another food. This may have you worried that they are malnourished. Don't worry, they are okay.

Yet another characteristic of toddler's eating patterns are mood swings that have them gorging one day and eating nothing the next. If you are unsure of how much your toddler should be eating per day to stay healthy, aim for between 75–90 calories per kilogram of body weight or 1,000 to 1,300 calories a day.[33]

You should avoid making little bargains with your child as in "one more bite and then you can have dessert". This causes the child to see the food as a way of bargaining with others emotionally and can lead to eating disorders later in life. The child may decide to use food as a reward or as a substitute for comfort.

One of the worst things you can do is force your child to eat. It teaches your child to rely on others to tell them what to eat and what they are thinking or feeling. This does not lead to healthy eating habits or good self-esteem.[34]

How to Get a Toddler to Eat Well

The difference between a baby and a toddler is that toddlers start to eat with their hands. This can start as early as eight months and it is the main activity of busy eaters; they love to explore, make a mess, and play with their foods.

The best thing to serve a grabby, curious little toddler is finger foods. Finger foods offer you the perfect opportunity to get your child familiar with eating things that have great nutrition. Furthermore, toddlers will develop a positive attitude towards food if they can look forward to eating fun foods at mealtime.

Here is a list of nutritious finger foods for toddlers that also amuse and delight them, so mealtime is a pleasure.

Fruit Slices: Arrange slices of his or her favourite fruits in a pinwheel or flower shape. An older toddler can cut shapes out of thin slices of melon, apples, or pears using small cookie cutters.

Dusty Snacks: Take diced banana, peach, avocado, cubed tofu, or other little cut-up foods and coat them with ground up wholewheat biscuit or wheatgerm.

Frozen Fruit Pops: On a hot day, these are perfect healthy treats. Cut up strawberries, pineapple, or bananas and stuff those into ice block moulds (little paper cups work, too). Fill with orange or another 100 percent juice, add ice block sticks, and freeze.

Vegetable Slices: These are harder to get a toddler to eat. Poaching and chilling the vegetables may help. Some babies like the feel of cold broccoli against their gums when they are teething.

It also helps to get creative with your foods. One great idea from paediatrician Dr. William Sears, suggests you put a variety of interesting foods in a large ice cube tray and present them to the baby.

Ideas for these foods are:

- Apple moons—thinly sliced
- Avocado boats—quarter of an avocado
- Broccoli trees—steamed broccoli
- Carrot swords—slivers of carrots
- Egg canoes—wedges of egg

- Cut up wedges of pancake

Allow your child to get as interactive with the food as possible. One way is to allow him or her to get messy by dipping vegetables or fruits. Use:

- Cottage cheese puree
- Whipped cream cheese
- Natural, organic preserves
- Guacamole (pureed avocado)
- Yogurt

If the child is not eating or is acting really stubborn, you can also make him or her a baby smoothie in the blender. Mix frozen fruits with yogurt for a tasty treat.[35]

It can also be a bit of a challenge to get a toddler to eat his or her vegetables. Some ideas for getting around this problem are:

- Slip grated or diced vegetables into rice, cottage cheese, and macaroni and cheese
- Camouflage them in a favourite sauce
- Make veggie art such as vegetable faces out of bits of vegetables

As is true with infants, beware of foods that are choking hazards, such as grapes, peanuts and tree nuts, chunky peanut butter, cherry tomatoes, popcorn, and chewing gum. It is best not to let them have these foods until after age four.[36]

Most toddlers want to get on a program where they are eating with the adults. Offer child-size utensils and provide help when needed so the child does not get frustrated when eating.

- Offer foods that can be picked up, chewed or gummed, and swallowed easily. (Be sure to watch your child closely and avoid foods that are choking hazards.)
- Make the meals about connecting with the child emotionally.
- Point and say the names of foods and make eating a learning project that you are enjoying together.
- Talk about things that you did that day to teach the child how to socialise.

It is okay to offer your child a healthy snack between meals, if you think he or she is hungry. Hunger can force your child to think that stuffing oneself is the answer.

It is an excellent idea to turn off the television, radio or other distractions while your toddler is eating. This helps the child focus on just eating food.[37]

Top Ten Tips for Feeding Toddlers

1. Invest in a good bib, many towels, and a mat for the floor. No matter what you do, the toddler is not going to be neat or tidy.
2. Whether making your own baby food or buying it, steer clear of the additives, pesticides, preservatives, and other toxic things described in Chapter 2 about feeding infants—all of the same principles apply to feeding a toddler.
3. Make sure your toddler is well hydrated, as they have more of a need to drink water than an infant who gets plenty of hydration from breast milk.

4. Don't feed your child too much juice; even the natural sugar in juices can give your child a mood swing that results in a high and then a terrible 'crash' or low mood.

5. Watch out for foods that are choking hazards like grapes, cherry tomatoes, and peanuts.

6. Do not use food as a bargaining chip or reward. Your child may start thinking that eating is a goal or some sort of emotional soothing. This can lead to a poor relationship with food later in life.

7. Do not shame or guilt your child while he or she is eating, or mealtimes may be associated with stress. This can also create an eating disorder later in life.

8. Keep mealtimes for your toddler under twenty minutes. They have short attention spans and there is no sense in keeping them in a chair to have a big ego struggle.

9. Encourage your toddler to play with his or her food. Invest in plastic cookie cutters so he or she can make shapes out of bread and other soft foods. This helps him or her develop a positive attitude towards mealtime.

10. Accept inconsistency. A toddler will gorge one day and then eat almost nothing the next. They also like to binge on one particular food for days. Do not be alarmed. This is normal temperamental toddler behaviour.

Chapter 4: Play Age Eating Patterns

(4–9 Years Old)

Play Age Eating Patterns

The play age years are also known as the "middle age of childhood" or the pre-adolescent years. You will notice that your child is going to be more interested in making choices when it comes to eating. Most children will display definite preferences for either one food or another.

These are also the years when you can really establish eating patterns that will function as the bedrock of health for your child's future years.

At this age, you'll notice your child is also more vulnerable to messages from the media and pressure from their peers to eat things that are unhealthy. The constant television commercials alone can make it difficult for a play age child to resist sugary, fatty, or refined foods.

At the same time, you might also notice that your child is more interested in learning about shopping and cooking. This offers you the ideal opportunity to teach them how to take care of their nutritional needs and enjoy what they make for themselves at mealtimes.

Eating patterns of these school-age children are now also destined to be somewhat out of your control, so it is important to educate them about what is best for them to eat when they are not at home.

The Play Age Eating Schedule

Children aged four to nine years old need to eat three sit-down square meals a day and at least three snacks a day.

It is important to control your child's diet from home. Regular home-cooked meals can help promote healthy eating habits. And don't forget that limiting your child's intake of fast foods and other unhealthy foods is a great way to control your child's intake of cholesterol.

Studies have shown that children who eat healthy meals at home are more likely to choose healthy snacks outside the home. That means saying 'no' to greasy chips and sugary cakes and lollies.

You should also pack your child's lunch. If your child must buy lunch, then make sure he or she can make the right food choices. Even very young children can be taught how to order healthy choices or shop for healthy groceries.

Special Nutritional Needs of Pre-Adolescents

In 2011, the nutritional needs of pre-adolescents, along with all other age groups and adults, were re-established as an initiative of Michelle Obama. The United States Department of Agriculture (USDA) replaced the traditional 19-year-old food pyramid with the My Plate[38] pictogram as a means of educating the public regarding dietary guidelines.

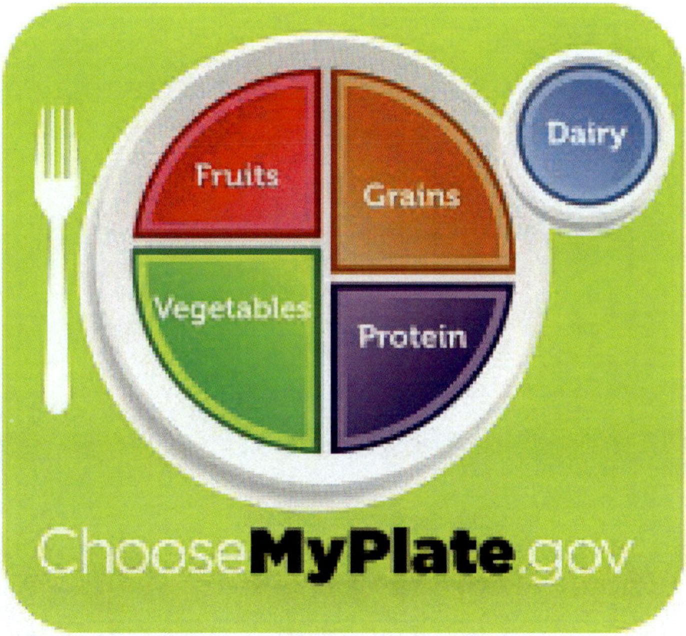

Instead of Meat, Dairy, Breads/Grains, and Fruits/Vegs, the four groups are now defined as *Fruits, Vegetables, Grains,* and *Proteins,* with a smaller group, *Dairy,* off to the side. Based on these food groups, the My Plate food guide is grouped according to five colours and focuses above all on nutrition and variety.

In Australia, we have the following recommendations with slightly different percentages.

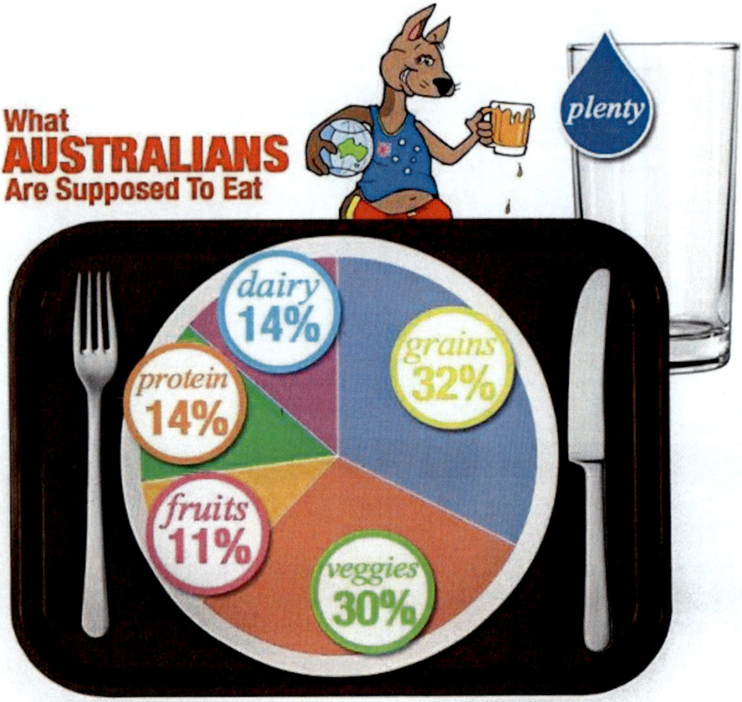

Source: www.eatforhealth.gov.au (Used with permission)

For more detail on the recommended foods, check out the complete diagram in the **Appendix**.

The amount of food a child should eat from each food group on a daily basis is determined by their age, sex, and physical activity level.

Grains: 32% (US 30%)

At best, all of your children's intake of grains should come from wholegrain sources, such as whole-wheat pasta and wholegrain rice. These types of grains contain complex carbohydrates that sustain energy over a number of hours.

Four- to eight-year-olds require about a half-cup serving of grains a day.

Vegetables: 30% (US 40%)

Children should consume a variety of different vegetables, especially different-coloured vegetables. They are a great source of vitamins, minerals, and phytonutrients that can't be found in other foods, and will boost the immune system. Vegetables are also an excellent source of fibre for children.

Buy or grow organic if you can. The healthier the soil, the more minerals the plant will take up and deliver to you and your child.

Children four to eight years old should have 1–1½ cups of vegetables daily.

Fruit: 11% (US 10%)

Fruit are also a great source of vitamins and phytonutrients, which help build the immune system.

Apples, berries, oranges, avocados, and peaches are all great choices, but any fruit your child likes is a good choice. Beware of giving too much fruit, however, because many fruits contain high amounts of natural sugar.

Children four to eight years old should have 1–1½ cups of fruit per day.

Protein: 14% (US 20%)

Meat is an important source of iron, which provides children with the energy they need on a daily basis. Opt for lean choices for your children's diet, such as skinless chicken and turkey.

Eggs are another great protein food. Most kids will eat omelettes or scrambled eggs, or you can add them to other dishes such as quiche.

Children between the ages of four to eight should have approximately 100 grams of protein daily,

Dairy 14%

We have more calcium in our bodies than any other mineral, and milk can be a good source. But milk can cause sensitivities or allergic reactions in many children, so opt for organic or pastured products; or try goat's milk, which contains less allergenic proteins and is easier to digest. Yogurt, low-fat cheese, and calcium-fortified orange juice are also great substitutes for milk and add variety to your child's diet.

It may be challenging, however, to get your child to consume enough calcium. Calcium helps ensure the proper formation of bones and teeth, and aids in heart and muscle function.

The Australian Dietary Guidelines outline how much calcium your child should be getting, depending upon his/her age.

Children four to eight years old should have 1–2 servings of milk or other dairy products a day.

One serving might look like:

- One cup (250 ml) glass of milk
- One 50-gram piece of cheese
- Three quarters of a cup of yogurt

While dairy products tend to be the best source of calcium for young children, it is not always possible to offer these food items to your child. If your child is allergic to cow's milk protein, or is vegan, you will need to find an alternative source of calcium. Some great foods high in calcium include:

- rice milk
- dark green leafy vegetables (cabbage leaves, kale, spinach, and bok choy)
- broccoli
- canned salmon with bones
- enriched fruit juices and fortified cereals
- soy products (but some children may have an allergic reaction; opt for organic non-GMO soy products)
- oranges

Unfortunately, calcium isn't always absorbed efficiently in your child's stomach. Vitamin D is essential for proper calcium absorption. 200 IUs of Vitamin D every day will help calcium be absorbed in the gastrointestinal tract, ensuring that your child gets the most out of his or her calcium intake.

Vitamin D is produced by the body when it is exposed to sunlight, especially during the warmer months of the year. Encourage your child to be active outdoors during this time period.

Vitamin D is found almost exclusively in animal products, so if your child can't get enough sunlight, these foods are high in Vitamin D:

- egg yolks
- cold-water fish (salmon, tuna)
- mushrooms
- fortified foods (soy products, orange juice, cereals)

Does your child ignore foods with calcium in them? Here are some suggestions for upping the calcium intake in everyday foods.

- Try adding flavour to a glass of milk. Chocolate or pureed fruit (strawberry and even banana) can make milk or yogurt more appealing. If you use store-bought syrup, look for syrups with little sugar and no additives.
- Sprinkle some cheese on top of vegetables or add a light cheese sauce or melted cheese over vegetables.
- Make soups and warm cereals with milk instead of water. This is a great way to sneak some extra calcium into your children's diet.
- Add home-made ice cream or yogurt to a variety of different fruits. You can make your own high-quality yogurt, and you can find recipes for home-made ice cream in my *Kids Love Ice Cream* book at **www.bestfoodfriends.com**.

This will not only increase your child's calcium intake, but it will also encourage him or her to develop a taste for healthy foods.

Here's a quick and easy recipe for yogurt bark.

Spread an approximately half a centimetre (1/4 inch) layer on a parchment paper-covered cookie sheet. Add toppings such as unsweetened shredded coconut, chopped nuts, diced fruits, or mini-chocolate chips. Pat toppings into yogurt and place in the freezer for 4 hours, then break into pieces. (Yogurt bark will turn soft quickly, so is not suitable for lunch boxes.)

School-age children need to eat the same healthy foods adults eat, along with more vitamins and minerals to support their growing bodies. This means whole grains (whole wheat, oats, barley, rice, millet, quinoa), a wide variety of fresh fruits and vegetables, calcium for growing bones (milk, yogurt or substitutes if lactose intolerant), and healthy proteins (fish, eggs, poultry, lean meat, nuts and seeds).

Healthy fats are also important at this age. There are two types that your child should be consuming.

- Monounsaturated fats: from plant oils like peanut oil and olive oil, as well as avocados, nuts (almonds, hazelnuts, and pecans), and seeds (pumpkin, sesame).
- Polyunsaturated fats: including Omega-3 and Omega-6 fatty acids found in fatty fish (salmon, herring, mackerel, anchovies, and sardines) or in unheated sunflower, corn, soybean, and flaxseed oils, and walnuts.

Children, like the rest of us, should limit trans fats that are found in vegetable shortenings, some margarine, crackers, lollies, biscuits and cookies, snack foods, fried foods, baked goods, and other processed foods made with partially hydrogenated vegetable oils.[39]

Issues and Challenges of Feeding Play Age Children

Children aged four to nine tend to develop the same types of unhealthy eating habits that adults do.

Many children have a hectic schedule and tend to gulp down food and eat too fast. This is why it is so important for you to establish regular mealtimes and take away all distractions during that mealtime so that the focus is eating the meal.

Studies have shown that children eating in front of the television or computer tend to eat mindlessly. They eat too much, and this leads to weight gain. Teach the child to sit down and share a meal with the family and avoid using the television as a "dinner time babysitter".

Children of this age also end up skipping meals for all kinds of reasons. This can happen at school, if you do not supply your child's lunch. Freeze meals ahead and instruct your child how to prepare them if you are not home in time for dinner.

Most kids like sugar and they will go to great lengths to get it. It makes them feel energetic and "high". Don't let your child make "any time" dessert time.

Speaking of sugar, do everything you can to avoid having your child become addicted to soft drinks. These sugary liquids play havoc with your child's blood glucose levels.

Limiting salt is also a big issue with children. One teaspoon contains 2,300 mg of sodium, which is ALL that a child much older (14 to 18 years old) should have. A child four to nine years old should only have 1,900 mg a day.[40]

You can help by preparing meals from scratch. Industrially processed foods, the kind that comes in boxes, cans, and packages, is generally high in sodium (frozen pizzas, burritos and tacos, lunch meats, canned soups and vegetables, snack foods, prepared foods).

The salt we buy in—table salt—is not natural salt and contains anti-caking agents. They're deemed safe, but natural salt (pink salt, grey salt, sea salt) contains 81 trace minerals.

On the down side, natural salt does not contain added iodine. If you opt for natural salt as a way to reduce sodium intake, make sure your kids are getting iodine from other sources (seafood: fish, sea vegetables).

Another issue when it comes to children is the school lunch. School lunches get boring for both parents and children and they end up taking lunch money to school instead of a lunch made at home.

Serving your child a well-balanced diet that includes all the food groups, as well as the occasional treat, sets the stage for your child to make the right choices later on.

Sometimes, children will take a lunch to school and then just not eat it. If this is the case, then make the lunch in front of the child. Be sure to give him or her choices of healthy options as you make it. It's likely he or she will tell you what they feel like eating and actually consume it at lunchtime. If your child plays a part in designing his or her own lunch, they will be less likely to spend money on junk food in the school cafeteria.

Here are some ideas for making school lunches more exciting:

- Pack exotic fruits like Japanese apple, or a blood orange, or dried fruits to create interest
- Include low-fat cheese or cheese sticks

- Veggies and pitta bread with a low-fat healthy vegetable-based dip can replace a salty bag of chips from the supermarket
- A box of raisins is a healthy treat
- Home-made rice pudding
- A 100-gram bar of dark chocolate (75–80% cocoa) contains heart-healthy antioxidants, 11 grams of fibre, helps control appetite, and promotes digestion[41]
- Add organic preserves or chopped tomatoes in olive oil for a tasty treat
- Make your own soup and send it along with your child in a thermos to keep it warm

The health food and grocery industry is becoming increasingly aware of the public's need to supply more nutritious foods for children for lunch, so keep your eye out for new products that are free of preservatives in the future.

Note: Remember fat-free and low-fat have many artificial ingredients—home-made is always best.

How to Get a Play Age child to Eat Healthy

Children get bored and you have to keep their meals interesting. Make sure your child's daily calorie intake is right for his or her age and activity.

Be sure to try new recipes and new healthy food products to add variety to your child's meals. The more creative you are in your cooking, the more likely your child is to enjoy eating it.

You may not be able to completely limit your child's intake of fat outside of the home, but whenever you can, be sure to use healthy oils, like olive to cook with instead of solid fats like butter. If you like the taste of butter (and who doesn't), buy pastured butter (from grass-fed animals) to limit the amount of pesticides found in animal feed (Westgold butter is an example of grass-fed butter).

Cooking with coconut oil is also highly recommended. It has high-temperature-heat resistance and will not form dangerous aldehydes, which are mutagenic and can cause genetic toxicity. This is particularly important when deep frying, something kids love (think French fries).

One way to start teaching children between four and nine years old how to eat right, is to take them grocery shopping with you. This gives you the opportunity to teach them healthy food buying habits that will stay with them for life. It may take you longer to shop, but it's worth the time and trouble.

While shopping you can teach children:

- How each item belongs to a food group
- Which foods can be consumed often, and which are occasional treats
- How to buy inexpensive fresh or frozen food
- How to read ingredient labels
- How to watch out for foods that are too high in calories; which foods have good calories, and which have empty calories
- How to avoid foods that have a list of ingredients that are too long or complicated (evidence that the product contains too many additives)

As kids get older, they'll learn more and understand more about reading food labels. The good shopping habits that you teach them now will last for a lifetime. These habits can include: avoiding impulse shopping, planning meals ahead for the week, and sticking to only buying things that are on a shopping list.

Other healthy eating tips you can teach your children include:

- Substituting soft drinks and sugary drinks with teas (hot or iced), home-made lemonades, and water
- Buying wholegrain breads instead of white
- Limiting the use of rich sauces like cheese or cream sauces
- Make eating fish three times a week a regular thing
- Choosing lean meat instead fatty meat
- Avoiding prepared foods with a high fat or high salt/sodium content
- You can also teach your children to cook using healthy foods that can be augmented with fresh toppings. Examples are pizza, tacos and quesadillas

Persuading your child to eat more fruits and vegetables may be more difficult as they get older because they are going to have more access to junk food than ever before.

Here are some ways to get more fruits and vegetables into his or her diet:

- Put bananas, apples, blueberries, or raisins in cereal
- Make frozen fruit kebabs out of chunks of fresh fruit
- Teach your child how to make a smoothie, or make them one full of fresh fruit as an afternoon snack
- Add vegetables and fruits to pancakes
- Make healthy cakes like carrot cakes or zucchini bread
- Make fun kebabs with grilled fruit and veggie chunks

Finally, getting children at this age to eat vegetables is all about ease and availability. If they can reach for a little bundle of celery and carrot sticks with a dip as easily as they can a bag of potato chips, then you have won half the battle. Keep crudités (cut up vegetables) ready and easy for your child to consume at any time.

Best Food Friends have a series of recipe books that have made it easier for parents to get their kids to eat healthy.

We have enlisted the help of a chef to prepare healthy versions of foods kids love to eat.

Kids Love Snacks
Kids Love Ice Cream
Kids Love Dips
Kids Love Pasta
Kids Love Pizza

Find out more about these books at
www.bestfoodfriends.com

Top Ten Tips for Feeding Play Age Children

1. Pack your child's lunch instead of giving him or her lunch money to make sure he or she has a nutritious midday meal.
2. School-age children don't eat as many vegetables as they should, so try and sneak as much into their diets as you can by adding extra vegetables and fruits to baked goods, soups and stews.
3. Keep cut-up vegetables and dips in the refrigerator ready for them to eat.

4. Eat fish three times a week to keep your child's brain healthy.

5. Instead of ice cream, serve them pops made from fruits, or smoothies made from blended frozen fruit.

6. Do not let your child eat too much salt. Avoid feeding them canned, packaged, and processed foods.

7. Teach your child how to make a shopping list and plan healthy foods for the week.

8. Ban soft drinks from your home; offer hot or cold teas, home-made lemonade and water instead.

9. Take your kids shopping with you and teach them to read nutritional labels so they know they're eating low-fat, nutrition-packed, and additive-free foods.

10. Teach them early in life how to make salads, tacos, pizzas, and other foods that require fresh ingredients so they will always be eating fresh vegetables.

Chapter 5: Pre-teen Eating Patterns

(10–13 Years Old)

Pre-teen Eating Patterns

Pre-teen eating patterns are similar to those in the pre-adolescent years. The good news is that pre-teens are at the optimum age to learn and retain information about nutrition and cooking healthy meals for themselves.

You might notice that they get a little pickier when it comes to food. In girls, this can have to do with being worried about their body image and trying to behave like a supermodel or actress they've seen on television.

According to many experts, all you need to do is make the meals nutritious and serve them on schedule. It is up to the teen to make the decision whether or not to eat them. Often the teen will eat if you do not monitor him or her too closely, as at this age they may be trying to assert independence from you simply by doing the opposite of what you tell them.

Not all pre-teens are picky. Many of them are interested in learning how to shop and cook to help out the family or simply because they enjoy exploring the culinary arts.

- Pre-teens (like play age children) will display definite likes and dislikes when it comes to food.
- They are often tempted by junk food due to being surrounded by messages from the media that make sugary, fatty, or refined foods, look delicious.

- They need to avoid snacking mindlessly between meals while watching television.

Like play age children, pre-teens are destined to be somewhat out of your control, so it is important to educate them about what is best for them to eat when they are not at home.

One characteristic that your child might start to display at this age is comfort eating. This is because a child this age may not know how to effectively cope with approaching puberty, hormones, feelings about the opposite sex, and many other pre-pubescent issues and emotions.

The Pre-teen Eating Schedule

Children from ages ten to thirteen years need to eat three sit-down square meals, and at least three snacks a day to stay healthy. However, some of these children may experience a big growth spurt that requires them to constantly be snacking. This is okay as long as the child is not gaining a great deal of weight, and as long as he or she is snacking on healthy foods. They will likely need higher-calorie foods to maintain growth spurts, so supply things like avocados, bananas, cheeses, raw nuts, and gluten-free, wholegrain crackers; add coconut oil to smoothies.

Most preteens are happiest eating three meals a day. Studies have shown that children who eat healthy meals at home with the family are more likely to choose healthy snacks outside the home. That means saying 'no' to many snack junk foods.[42]

Like play age children, your preteen is vulnerable to the temptations at local fast food outlets and has more expendable income of his or her own.

If your child must buy lunch, then make sure he or she can make the right food choices. One way to control how your adolescent spends money on food is to give them a prepaid debit card; this will give you a good idea of how much they are eating, when they are eating, and what they are buying.

Special Nutritional Needs of Pre-teens

The nutritional needs of pre-teens are almost identical to the guidelines for eating outlined in the Chapter 4: 'Play Age Eating Patterns'.

In summary, pre-teens need to:

- Eat regularly
- Stay away from junk food
- Avoid excess salt and sugar
- Make sure they are getting enough calcium through food sources
- Make sure they are getting enough Vitamin D from food and sunlight.

Feed your child based on the Australian Guidelines for Healthy Eating and make sure that:

- Half of your children's intake of carbohydrates is from grains and that boys are getting 150 grams and girls are getting 175 grams
- A variety of vegetables are consumed as a source of vitamins and fibre, with girls over ten needing 2 cups of vegetables a day and boys over ten needing 2½ cups of vegetables

- Girls and boys over ten should have between 1 and 1½ cups of fruit a day
- Both boys and girls should have three servings of dairy products every day
- Boys and girls both need 150 grams of meat per day

As is true with younger children, pre-teens may not be getting enough calcium, which helps ensure the proper formation of bones and teeth. Children between the ages of ten and nineteen should be getting at least 1,300 milligrams of calcium every day.

Children who are allergic to cow's milk protein, or who are vegan, will need to find an alternative source of calcium. Some great foods high in calcium include cheese, soy milk, rice milk, salmon, broccoli, and fortified foods (orange juice and cereals).

Vitamin D is essential for proper calcium absorption. 200 IUs of Vitamin D every day will help calcium be absorbed in the gastrointestinal tract, ensuring that your child gets the most out of their calcium intake.

As school-age children develop, they need more vitamins and minerals to support their growing bodies. This means whole grains (whole wheat, oats, barley, rice, millet, quinoa), a wide variety of fresh fruits and vegetables, calcium for growing bones (milk, yogurt, or substitutes) and healthy proteins (fish, eggs, poultry, lean meat, nuts, and seeds).

Healthy fats are also important at this age as the brain is developing. There are two types that your child should be consuming.

- Monounsaturated fats: from plant oils like peanut oil and olive oil, as well as avocados, nuts, and seeds

- Polyunsaturated fats: including Omega-3 and Omega-6 fatty acids, found in fish such as salmon, herring, mackerel, anchovies, and sardines, or in unheated sunflower, corn, soybean and flaxseed oils, and raw walnuts

Pre-adolescents should also avoid food that contains vegetable shortenings and trans fats, which are included in some types of margarine, most crackers, lollies, biscuits and cookies, snack foods, fried foods, baked goods, and other processed foods made with hydrogenated or partially hydrogenated vegetable oils. Manufacturers use them to increase shelf life and they have no nutritional value, but they do a lot of harm.[43]

A word on saturated fats: A worldwide study of fat intake (See Endnote 43), revealed that people outside the US, who ate the most saturated fat, had a 21% lower risk for stroke. This is likely due to the fact that people around the world, outside the US, pasture their animals. These animals are not raised in confined feeding operations, so their fat is healthy, not filled with the toxins, pesticides, steroids, and added hormones that are put into the feed used in concentrated animal feeding operations.[44]

The brain needs fat. Don't eliminate saturated fat from your kid's diet completely. Get good clean saturated fat from grass-fed animals and their products.

Pre-teen Feeding Challenges and Issues

Children aged ten to twelve are in a lot of danger of developing unhealthy eating habits. To prevent them from doing things like gulping food, you need to make sure that the focus is on eating the meal.

Pre-teens have all of the feeding challenges and issues that younger play age children do including:

- Mindlessly eating in front of the television
- Skipping meals to socialise or because of emotional upsets
- Eating poorly in school cafeterias
- Getting addicted to sugar.

For more tips about how to nip these bad habits in the bud, read the 'Play Age Eating Patterns' section in Chapter 4.

This is also an age at which your child might start to show signs of an eating disorder. This is more prevalent in teenagers, but be wary of such behaviours as:

- Stopping eating and drinking
- Talking constantly about being skinny
- Being secretive or dismissive about food intake
- Developing strange eating habits like pushing the food around the plate and never consuming it
- Vomiting after eating
- Losing a great deal of weight.

If you suspect your pre-teen is too obsessed with his or her weight, get professional advice immediately. Eating disorders can result in everything from tooth loss to organ damage to brain damage, and they have the best recovery results if treated early.[45]

Persuading Your Pre-teen to Eat Well

Like play age children, pre-teen children get bored, so you have to keep their meals interesting. Make sure your child's daily calorie intake is right for his or her age and activity.

Try new recipes and new healthy food products to help add variety to your child's meals. The more creative and contemporary you are in your cooking, the more likely your child is going to like eating it.

Many of the same persuasion techniques described in the previous chapter on play age children also apply here as well.

To persuade your pre-teen to eat well:

- Take them grocery shopping with you to learn how to buy nutritional wholesome foods and stick to a grocery list
- Instil the "never shop when you are hungry" rule
- Teach them how to read ingredient labels
- Substitute soft drinks with teas, home-made lemonades and water
- Buy wholegrain breads, pastas, and rice
- Encourage eating more fish
- Teach them how to buy lean meats
- Encourage them to cook healthy foods like home-made pizza and tacos
- Add more fruit to cereals
- Drink more smoothies full of vegetable or fruit combinations
- Make healthy cakes out of zucchini, chia, and carrots.

Finally, getting kids of this age to eat vegetables is all about access. Be sure to have healthy food readily accessible in the home for your child to consume at any time.

One common issue that often comes up at this age is that of vegetarianism. Children who are ten to twelve can become very concerned with the environment and treatment of animals.

Let your child know that you approve of his or her decision to become a vegetarian, but at the same time make sure you sit down and plan a diet with your child.

Vegetarian diets can be missing protein, iron, Vitamin B12 and calcium, so be sure to provide supplementation if needed. You should also be aware that a vegetarian child may gain weight a lot quicker simply because they tend to eat less protein and more foods high in carbohydrates like grains and breads. (See Endnote 44.)

One thing that might work for you is getting your child to "Colour Their Diet". This teaches them to eat the dark and richly coloured vegetables that are so good for them:

- Brown foods include: whole grains like mahogany rice or whole-wheat bread, figs, brown pears, walnuts, cinnamon, kidney beans, and spelt noodles.
- Black foods include lentils, black soybeans, and blackberries.
- Beige and white foods include: white beans, chickpeas, cauliflower, bananas, and sweet onions.
- Red foods include: pomegranates, raspberries, red quinoa, beetroot, cherries, and rhubarb.
- Yellow foods include: pineapples, squash, and star fruit. Try whole-wheat spaghetti in place of white, refined spaghetti for added fibre.
- Blue foods include blueberries and plums.

- Purple foods include eggplant, red cabbage (which looks purple), blood oranges (which can be purple inside), and purple potatoes.
- Green foods include: avocado, silver beet, broccoli, coriander, sugar snap and other peas, Brussel sprouts, and kiwi fruits.
- Orange foods include: mangos, carrots, oranges, pumpkin, orange baby tomatoes, sweet potato, and apricots.

The idea is to eat at least eight different colours a day to stay healthy.[46]

Instead of having the media work against you, you can use sources of information online to educate your pre-adolescent. The following are some good sites for children between ten and thirteen to explore.

www.empowerme2be.com

This site helps motivate kids to be healthier by joining in polls and forums. It also offers practical tips for parents. It is run by the Alliance for a Healthier Generation.

www.nourishinteractive.com

Nurses and registered dietitians run this energetic site teeming with online games for kids, plus blogs, newsletters, health-hint calendars, lesson plans, and worksheets for parents and educators.

www.kidsyogastories.com

Children visiting this site will find 58 yoga poses for kids, as well as, stories from other kids around the world. It encourages healthy eating and physical activity.

www.kidnetic.com

Find more games here, plus recipes and other content offered by the International Food Information Network Solutions Group.

www.superkidsnutrition.com

This is a great site full of tools, books, resources and recipes that cater to younger kids. There are articles about cooking and gardening for young kids, too.

Top Ten Tips for Feeding Pre-teens

1. If your child is picky about eating food, realise that it might be more about you than the food as ego struggles are likely at this age. Patience and non-resistance are key.
2. Do not be surprised if your child is a binge eater or craves one particular food. As long as it's not an unhealthy food, you should indulge the craving.
3. Train your child to eat eight servings of antioxidant-laden fruits and vegetables a day by eating by colour.
4. Do not be surprised if your pre-teen starts talking about becoming a vegetarian; this is a "hot topic" around the first decade of life and should be encouraged as long as your child gets all of the vitamins they need in supplements (especially B12).
5. Discourage your pre-teen from being an emotional eater. Explain how food should not be used to abate extreme feelings or avoid dealing with reality.
6. Be aware of the signs of anorexia and bulimia and get your pre-teen professional help quickly if you suspect body-image issues. Even though these disorders are associated with teenagers, they can start at a very young age.

7. Reward your child if they resist the temptation to eat in the school cafeteria and take a home-made lunch to school instead.

8. Continue to take your child shopping and encourage him or her to read nutritional labels and try new foods.

9. Encourage your child to cook meals for the family; in some communities, you might be able to enrol your child in a cooking and nutrition class. Usually these types of classes advertise through extended education brochures and local newspapers.

10. Your child can read and learn from online sources at this point, so be sure to take advantage of interactive tools on the internet that might encourage him or her to pay more attention to their health.

Chapter 6: Teen Eating Patterns

(13–19 Years Old)

What to Expect from an Adolescent

When your child hits age thirteen, you can expect a noticeable growth spurt. The nutritional needs of your child are greatly increased because of the changes in body composition and increased growth rate that is associated with sexual development and puberty.

Some teens do not change a lot but most experience a dramatic need for all kinds of different foods. Many teens are also incredibly active and expend a lot of fuel. Many spend more time working either at a job or with increased work from school; they socialise more, exercise more and have more erratic behaviours in general that affect how and when they eat.[47]

Your Teen's Eating Schedule

In theory, a teenager needs three square meals a day and to eat several nutritious snacks a day to stay healthy and keep up with growth. However, most teens are as restless as they were when they were growing toddlers. That is because they are going through a major growth spurt.

For many different reasons it may be difficult to get your teenager to sit down with your family and eat a meal. However, this is crucial to getting some control over his or her diet.

One trick is to assign as a duty to your teen for them to cook dinner for the entire family a few days every week. That way the teen is occupied with matters to do with nutrition and has less time to eat junk after school. Yet another benefit to this approach is that it gives your adolescent an opportunity to feel accomplished in choosing healthy meals to cook for themselves and the whole family. You will also be giving your teenager healthy eating and cooking skills for life.

Special Nutritional Needs of a Teenager

US national and population-based surveys have found that adolescents often fail to meet dietary recommendations for overall nutritional status and for specific nutrient intakes.

During this age **emotional eating is prevalent**. Many crave sugar and fat and succumb to that temptation to gorge on junk food. This results in lower than the recommended intake of Vitamin A, folic acid, fibre, iron, calcium and zinc.

According to one study, the low intake of iron and calcium among adolescent girls is of particular concern. Iron deficiency can impair cognitive function and physical performance, and inadequate calcium intake may increase fracture risk during adolescence and the risk of developing osteoporosis in later life.[48]

If your adolescent seems stressed or sick, then take him or her to a doctor. The culprit could very well be a lack of nutrients in their diet.

For healthy adolescents, the following is recommended.

- Eat three meals a day, with healthy snacks in between.
- Increase fibre in their diet and decrease the use of salt and sugar.
- Drink plenty of water.

- For growing children and adolescents who need extra calories to keep up with growth spurts, it is generally recommended to limit the total healthy fat consumption to 35% of calories rather than counting calories.
- Eat well-balanced meals often.
- When cooking for your adolescent, try to bake, steam or boil instead of fry.
- Make sure your adolescent is not overdosing on sugar,
- Eat fruits or vegetables for snacks.
- Decrease the use of butter and heavy gravies.
- Eat more chicken and fish[49]

It is helpful for your teenager to eat following the Australian Dietary Guidelines.

Note that a lot of this advice has been covered before in previous chapters in this book, as solid common sense about dieting does not change from phase to phase in the growth of human development.

Adolescent Food Issues and Challenges

Healthy eating during adolescence is important as many body changes during this time affect an individual's nutritional and dietary needs.

Adolescents are becoming more independent and making many food decisions on their own.

They have many of the challenges that they have experienced earlier in life as a pre-teen but they are usually doubled in their frequency and intensity. Reading Chapters 4 and 5 (Play Age and Pre-teens) on getting enough vitamins and minerals can help you understand what your adolescent needs to eat to stay healthy.

Many adolescents experience a growth spurt around age thirteen, as well as an increase in appetite, and need healthy foods to meet their growth needs.

Adolescents tend to eat more meals away from home than younger children and are also heavily influenced by their peers, so as a parent, you must be aware of your adolescent's nutritional needs.

Be aware that a child that is not eating at all may have an underlying issue that is not food related. Nip these habits in the bud by addressing the matter directly as soon as you can as they are damaging to every aspect of your teenager's growth.

Two of the biggest food-related problems affecting teenagers are bulimia and anorexia. The list below explains these behavioural issues and illustrates how they can damage a young person in both mind and body.

Anorexia:

Although it usually afflicts adolescent girls, it is a behavioural disorder that can lead the individual to starve herself (or himself) in pursuit of an unrealistic body image. A potentially deadly disorder, anorexia impacts the self-image of the individual, as they look in the mirror and see someone ugly and overweight no matter how thin they actually are.[50]

Bulimia:

Bulimics will eat a large meal and then vomit or purge it so they do not absorb the calories and gain weight. Typically, the individual will go to the bathroom immediately following a meal and force themselves to vomit. Bulimia can be extremely harmful to the internal organs, teeth and functions of the developing teen. (See Endnote 50.)

Binge Eating

Some overweight teens (and indeed many who are not overweight) will engage in binge eating. This behaviour sees the individual consume large amounts of food compulsively as a response to stress or other "triggers" in their environment.

Constant vomiting can cause the acid in the stomach to damage the stomach lining and other internal organs. Binge eating can quickly lead to obesity, heart problems and a lack of overall health.

If this gets bad enough, you may have to place the teen into an Eating Disorders Program. (See Endnote 50.)

Warning Signs of Eating Disorders include:

- Being far too concerned about weight
- Strict dieting followed by high-calorie eating binges
- Overeating when distressed
- Feeling out of control
- Disappearing after a meal
- Depressed or antisocial behaviour
- Alcohol or drug abuse
- Frequent use of laxatives or diuretics
- Excessive exercising
- Irregular menstrual cycles

If your adolescent is showing any of these symptoms, it is time to intervene. The emotional and physical consequences of these disorders can last a lifetime. (See Endnote 50.)

Persuading Your Teenager to Eat Healthy

Meal convenience is important to many adolescents and this may lead them to eat too much of the wrong kinds of foods (e.g., soft drinks, fast-food, processed foods).

You can steer your teens around these matters by doing the following:

- Being sure that you have nutritious snacks always on hand.
- Don't give your adolescent any double messages, or they will think you are a hypocrite. Do not bring junk foods into your home for you to eat. Lead by example.
- Take their suggestions as to what they would like to eat and make low-fat versions of it—especially if it's junk food that can be modified like fried chicken or hamburgers.
- Vary their diets by cooking foods from other cultures such as Mexican, Indian or Chinese food (be sure to skip the MSG)[51]

Adolescents really need to steer away from any additives or foods containing added hormones since they may already be having enough problems with their body chemistry as they try to navigate puberty.

One thing that does work is to appeal to a teenager's vanity. They are very concerned with their appearance at this age so reminding them that eating healthy helps them to look good is a great idea.

Top Ten Tips for Feeding Teenagers

1. Do not tempt fate by bringing junk food for yourself or other family members into the home if you are trying to keep a teenager healthy.
2. Be aware that your teen might be short of some essential nutrients and may need supplementation with Vitamin A, folate, fibre, iron, calcium and zinc. (Look for supplements with "folate", not the synthetic version, "folic acid".)[52]
3. Most teenagers are quite concerned with their appearance and can be convinced that they will be slimmer and more attractive (i.e., clear skin, bright eyes, healthy hair) if they eat a healthy diet and exercise.
4. Make low-fat versions of junk food menu favourites; there are many recipes to be found online that can help you make healthy versions of junk food favourites like French fries, cheeseburgers, tacos and fried chicken.
5. Make food more interesting by cooking ethnic versions; this will help to keep your teen interested in mealtimes.
6. Curb cravings for junk foods by making sure that your teen is getting adequate supplementation with vitamins and minerals he or she may not be getting from food.
7. As was true with the pre-teen, keep your eye out for the warning signs and symptoms of eating disorders such as anorexia or bulimia and get them professionally treated if need be.

8. Never use food as a reward for good behaviour or have your teen associate it with love and affection; this can lead to eating disorders and poor self-esteem.

9. If your child is an emotional eater, intervene and educate him or her about their own personal triggers and how best to combat them without the need for emotional eating.

10. Be aware that a child who is not eating at all may have an underlying issue that is not food-related. Nip these habits in the bud by addressing the matter directly and without hesitation.

Conclusion: The Benefits of a Well-Nourished Child

The benefits of making sure that your child eats properly straight from birth to adulthood are countless.

Here is what you can accomplish for your child if you follow the advice in this book.

- An emotionally balanced individual who is less likely to suffer from mood swings or depression.
- A physically healthier person who is less prone to diseases of all kinds.
- A person who is not likely to develop allergies or other disorders.
- A person who is less prone to obesity.
- An individual who has a healthy self-image and does not need to resort to destructive behaviours like bulimia or anorexia.
- A calm, productive, and alert person who does well in school and work.
- A sensible, nutritionally educated adult who does not blow money on expensive junk food or impulse purchases at the grocery store.
- A person who can cook healthy nutritious meals and pass good lifestyle habits through to the next generation.

Above all, you will be raising an individual who is accountable for themselves and who is less likely to be a burden on the medical system.

Furthermore, your grandchildren are likely to be healthier as well. Good nutrition is a gift that keeps on giving for all of the people who have learned it, and are descended, from you.

Appendix

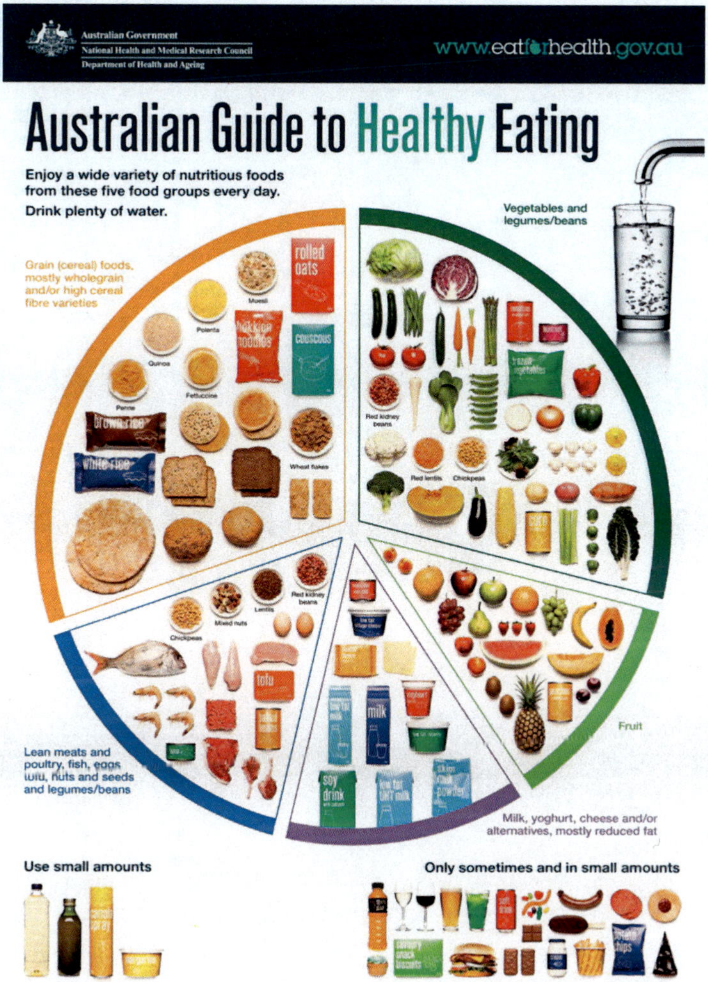

Source: www.eatforhealth.gov.au (Used with permission)

About the Author

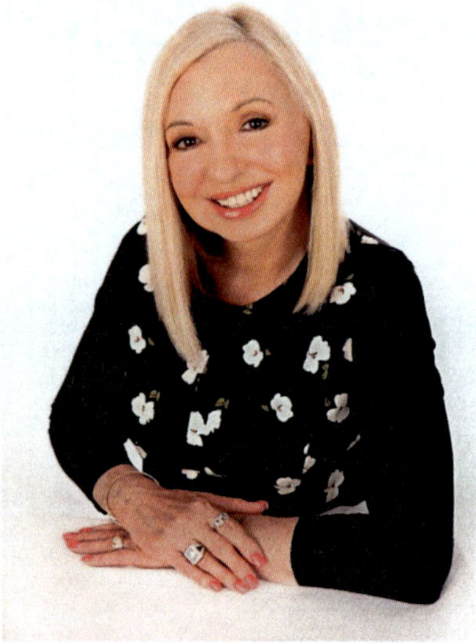

Catherine Chapman is a published author and is certified in childhood and adolescent nutrition (establishing healthy eating patterns for children and adolescents).

She is a certified personal trainer, a personal development coach and a holistic health coach. She is a graduate of the Institute of Integrative Nutrition (IIN) in New York and is published internationally with her Best Food Friends series of children's books.

References

[1] Mayo Clinic Staff. "Breast-feeding vs. formula-feeding. What's best?" Mayo Clinic: Healthy Lifestyle: Infant and toddler health. Mayo Foundation for Medical Education and Research, 2019. **https://www.mayoclinic.org/healthy-lifestyle/infant-and-toddler-health/in-depth/breast-feeding/art-20047898**

[2] Staff. "Breastfeed FAQs: How Much and How Often". Kids Health. Nemours, 2019.
https://kidshealth.org/en/parents/breastfeed-often.html

[3] Eidelman, Arthur I. MD and Schanler, Richard J. MD, et al. "Breastfeeding and the Use of Human Milk". AAP News & Journals Gateway. American Academy of Pediatrics' *Pediatrics*. March 2012, Volume 129 / Issue 3.

[4] Staff. "Things to Avoid When Breastfeeding". Healthy Children.org. American Academy of Pediatrics, 2009.

[5] Lerman, Y. et al. "Epidemiology of acute diarrheal diseases in children in a high standard of living rural settlement in Israel". Europe PMC. *The Pediatric Infectious Disease Journal*, 01 Feb 1994.
https://europepmc.org/abstract/med/8190536

[6] Sears, Dr. William P. "Benefits of Breastmilk". Ask Dr Sears. 2019. **https://www.askdrsears.com/topics/feeding-eating/breastfeeding/why-breast-is-best/benefits-of-breastmilk**

[7] Vennemann, M.M., et al. "Does Breastfeeding Reduce the Risk of Sudden Infant Death Syndrome?" AAP News & Journals Gateway. American Academy of Pediatrics' *Pediatrics*. March 2009, volume 123 / Issue 3.

[8] Betkowski, Bev. "How nursing mothers can help protect their babies from food allergies". Medical Xpress. University of Alberta, 17 July 2018

[9] Staff. "Can anything prevent my child from getting eczema?" American Academy of Dermatology. AAD, 2018.
https://www.aad.org/public/diseases/eczema/prevent-my-child-from-getting-eczema

[10] Lucas, Alan, et al. "Breast Milk and Subsequent Intelligence Quotient in Children Born Pre-Term". Article in *The Lancet* 339(8788):261-4. Research Gate, March 1992.

[11] Blacher, Brett, DDS. "3 Surprising Ways That Breast Milk Affects Your Child's Teeth". Pediatric Dentistry, 23 May 2018. **https://www.brettblacher.com/3-surprising-ways-that-breast-milk-affects-your-childs-teeth/**

[12] Martens, PJ, et al. "Breastfeeding Helps to Prevent Type 1 Diabetes". Diabetes in Control. Diabetesincontrol.com, 20 May 2017.
http://www.diabetesincontrol.com/breastfeeding-helps-to-prevent-type-1-diabetes/

[13] Stuebe, Allison, MD, MSc. "The Risks of Not Breastfeeding for Mothers and Infants". Obstetrics & Gynecology. U.S. National Library of Medicine National Institutes of Health, 2009.
https://www.ncbi.nlm.nih.gov/pmc/articles/PMC2812877/

[14] Staff. "How Can I Tell If My Baby is Eating Enough". Kids Health. Nemours, 1995.
http://kidshealth.org/parent/pregnancy_newborn/breastfeed/breastfeed_often.html#

[15] Mercola, Joseph, D.O. "Why You Should Embrace Healthful Sun Exposure". Mercola. Mercola.com, 11 Feb 2019.
https://articles.mercola.com/sites/articles/archive/2019/02/11/importance-of-sensible-sun-exposure.aspx

[16] Miller, Claire Cain and Carroll, Aaron E. "Should Your Baby Really Sleep in the Same Room as You?" The Upshot. *The New York Times*, 4 Nov 2016.
https://www.nytimes.com/2016/11/06/upshot/should-your-baby-really-sleep-in-the-same-room-as-you.html

[17] DuMond, Sara, MD. "An Age-by-Age Guide to Feeding Your Baby Solid Foods". Parents.com. *Parents Magazine*. Accessed 5 May 2019. **https://www.parents.com/baby/feeding/solid-foods/introducing-baby-to-solids/**

[18] Staff. "Why is Iron Important for Your Baby?" Parents.com *Parents Magazine*, Accessed 5 May 2019. **https://www.parents.com/baby/feeding/nutrition/why-iron-is-important/**

[19] Staff. "Solid foods: How to get your baby started". Healthy Lifestyle: Infant and toddler health. Mayo Clinic.org, 2019. **https://www.mayoclinic.org/healthy-lifestyle/infant-and-toddler-health/in-depth/healthy-baby/art-20046200**

[20] Staff. "Feeding Baby: How to Avoid Food Allergies". WebMD. WebMD, LLC. 2019. **https://www.webmd.com/parenting/baby/introducing-new-foods#1**

[21] Hull, Janet. Sweet Poison: How the World's Most Popular Artificial Sweetener is Killing Us. New Jersey: New Horizon Press, 1998.

[22] Scotti, Kelly, HHC. "The Dirty Dozen: 12 Food Additives to Avoid and Why". Food Democracy. 18 Jan 2008. **http://fooddemocracy.wordpress.com/2008/01/18/the-dirty-dozen-12-foodsfood-additives-to-avoid-and-why/**

[23] Baby Center Medical Advisory Board. "Foods That Can Be Unsafe For Your Baby". Baby Center 2011. **https://www.babycenter.com/0_foods-that-can-be-unsafe-for-your-baby_9195.bc**

[24] Baby Center Staff. "Pesticides in your child's food: What you need to know". Baby Center 2019.

[25] Admin. "Easy Homemade Baby Recipes". Wholesome Baby Food 2003. **http://www.wholesomebabyfood.com/**

[26] Baby Center Staff. "Introducing Solid Food: Solid Feeding Basics". Baby Center LLC 1997. **http://www.babycenter.com/0_introducing-solid-food_113.bc?page=2**

[27] Staff. "Introducing Solid Foods to Your Baby". Health Link BC. 2019. **https://www.healthlinkbc.ca/health-topics/te4473**

[28] Warnick, Melody. "Bye-Bye, Bottle". Parents.com. *Parents Magazine* June 2011 Issue. **https://www.parents.com/baby/breastfeeding/weaning/bye-bye-bottle/**

[29] Burritt, Kara. "Toddler Feeding Schedule: A Guide to Planning Meals". Parents.com **https://www.parents.com/toddlers-preschoolers/feeding/healthy-eating/toddler-feeding-schedule/**

[30] American Academy of Pediatrics Committee on Nutrition. "The Use and Misuse of Fruit Juice in Pediatrics". AAP News & Journals Gateway. *Pediatrics,* May 2001, volume 107 / Issue 5

[31] Vohra, Pankaj, Dr. "How Much Water Should My Toddler Drink Every Day?" Baby Center 2011. **https://www.babycenter.in/x1016988/how-much-water-should-my-toddler-drink-every-day**

[32] Staff. "What is Nitrate?" Centers for Disease Control and Prevention. U.S. Department of Health & Human Services, 2019. **https://www.cdc.gov/healthywater/drinking/private/wells/disease/nitrate.html**

[33] Staff. "How Much Does My Kid Need to Eat?" Parents.com. *Parents Magazine* 2018

[34] Gavin, Mary L. MD. "Toddlers at the Table: Avoiding Power Struggles". Kids Health. Nemours, 2019. **https://kidshealth.org/en/parents/toddler-meals.html**

[35] Sears, Dr. William P. "5 Ways to Use Yogurt as a Nutritious Substitute". Ask Dr Sears.com. **https://www.askdrsears.com/topics/feeding-eating/family-nutrition/yogurt/5-ways-use-yogurt-nutritious-substitute**

[36] Staff. "Tips to avoid a food choking hazard". Strong 4 Life. Children's Healthcare of Atlanta. 2019. **https://www.strong4life.com/en/pages/healthy-eating/articles/common-food-choking-hazards-and-how-to-avoid-them**

[37] Grogan, Alisha, MOT, OTR/L. "Why Screen Time and Eating are a Bad Idea". Your Kids Table. 2019. **https://yourkidstable.com/turn-off-tv/**

[38] United States Department of Agriculture - MyPlate Graphic Resources (converted from PDF), Public Domain, **https://commons.wikimedia.org/w/index.php?curid=38658432**

[39] Paul, Maya W. "Nutrition for Children and Teens". Help Guide. Help Guide International, 2011

[40] Staff. "Sea Salt vs. Table Salt". American Heart Association, 2019. **https://www.heart.org/en/healthy-living/healthy-eating/eat-smart/sodium/sea-salt-vs-table-salt**

[41] Bedwell, Sarah-Jane. "Dark Chocolate Contains a Shocking Amount of…" Self.com. Condé Nast, March, 2015. **https://www.self.com/story/dark-chocolate-contains-fiber**

[42] Staff. "Science says: eat with your kids". The Conversation. The Conversation US. Jan. 2015 **https://theconversation.com/science-says-eat-with-your-kids-34573**

[43] Cherney, Kristeen. "% Ways to Avoid Hydrogenated Oil". Healthline.com. Healthline Media, July 2018. **https://www.healthline.com/health/ways-to-avoid-hydrogenated-oil**

[44] Savedge, Jenn. "Massive food study puts current nutrition standards into question". MNN.com. Mother Nature Network, Sept. 2017. **https://www.mnn.com/food/healthy-eating/blogs/massive-food-study-puts-current-nutrition-standards-into-question**

[45] Mackenzie, Colleen. "Information for Preteens: Body Science About Eating Disorders". Sutter Health. Palo Alto Medical Foundation, 2013.

[46] Staff. "Eat More Color". American Heart Association. 2019. **https://www.heart.org/en/healthy-living/healthy-eating/add-color/eat-more-color**

[47] Oswalt, Angela, MSW. "Adolescent Physical Development". Mental Help.net. American Addiction Centers, Inc. 2019. **https://www.mentalhelp.net/articles/adolescent-physical-development/**

[48] Seiga-Riz, A.M., Carson T., Popkin B. "Three Squares or Mostly Snacks – what do teens really eat? A sociodemographic study of meal patterns". PubMed.gov Journal of Adolescent Health, 1998.
https://www.ncbi.nlm.nih.gov/pubmed/9436064

[49] Staff. "Healthy Eating During Adolescence". Johns Hopkins Medicine. Johns Hopkins University, 2019.
https://www.hopkinsmedicine.org/health/wellness-and-prevention/healthy-eating-during-adolescence

[50] Mayo Clinic Staff. "Teen eating disorders: Tips to protect your teen". Healthy Lifestyle Tween and Teen health. Mayo Clinic, 2019. **https://www.mayoclinic.org/healthy-lifestyle/tween-and-teen-health/in-depth/teen-eating-disorders/art-20044635**

[51] Zeratsky, Katherine, R.D., L.D. "What is MSG? Is it Bad for you?" Healthy Lifestyle Nutrition and healthy eating. Mayo Clinic, 2019.

[52] Arnarson, Atli, PhD. "Folic Acid vs Folate – What's the Difference?" Healthline. Healthline Media, 2019.
https://www.healthline.com/nutrition/folic-acid-vs-folate#section6

Made in United States
North Haven, CT
04 November 2026

21736088R00055